CONTENTS

INTRODUCTION

Air fryers are also among the best kitchen appliances on the market, second only to the Instant Pot. But these contrivances, usually serving only one purpose, eat up a considerable amount of valuable counter space. No wonder new products that aim to merge air fry technology with the conventional appliances that people already have in their kitchens have been reckless.

The latest entry, the Ninja Foodi Digital Air Fry Oven, incorporates an air fryer and toaster oven into one compact package to expand on the popularity of established Ninja Foodi products. But, is the investment worth it? We checked the Ninja Foodi oven to see if it would actually be able to merge two pieces of equipment into one without cheating on either.

You get a feeling as soon as you take it out of the box that the Foodi Digital Air Fry Oven is a high-quality product. Crafted of polished stainless steel, it is beautifully finished with rounded corners and has a digital pad for power. This is also larger than a standard toaster oven and narrower

The Foodi Oven can be turned on one side when cooled and not in use to stand up at the back of the table, an unusual yet convenient solution for storage. It has a tiny one off to the side you use to open the door, rather than a towel bar handle at the end. Although it's unique and takes some time to get used to it, this handle works very well and helps make the oven more effective in space.

The Foodi Digital Air Fry Oven comes complete with an air fry pot, a cooking rack, a non-stick sheet pan, and a crumb tray that also looks durable and well made. They are bigger than the ones you normally find in a toaster oven, because the oven is so wide.

BENEFITS OF DIGITAL AIR FRY OVEN

The digital air fry oven packs a lot of features and cooking capacity in a small countertop footprint. Air fry, air roast, air broil, bake, bagel, toast, dehydrate, and keep warm - all in one appliance - and when you're done cooking, reclaim your counter space by simply flipping the oven up and away to clean and store.

Pros
- Takes less space on the countertop
- Quiet operation
- Clear and easy to read control panel
- Very versatile
- Great value due to multi functions
- Cooks evenly
- Easy cleaning
- Preheats almost instantly, 60 seconds
- Easy Storage because of flip capabilities

Cons
- Cant cook full chicken
- Requires cleaning after every use
- Anti stick pan will warp at 400F
- Not enough space inside

Design

The design of the Ninja Foodi digital air fryer is well though to accommodate the multiple functions and still take less space on the countertop.

It takes 50% less space when flipped up and away to store against the backsplash.

The stainless steel construction makes the oven durable and looks sleek. Its color mixes black and stainless steel finish.

For large cooking purposes, it comes with a usable pan cooking area that can fit 13-inch pizza, up to 9 slices of toast and 6 chicken breasts.

Control Panel

Using the digital control panel of the air fryer oven is easy. The panel is well designed for clear and easy reading of the functions.

A knob is used to select the temperature and time for all the functions. Interior lights make it easy to monitor the progress inside and on the control panel.

Performance

Ninja's oven unique design and 1800 wattage enable faster cooking within 20 minutes. It takes 60 seconds to preheat to save time, unlike traditional ovens.

Digital Crisp Control Technology enables precisely controlled temperature and fan speeds for delicious results.

Air Roasting

Ninja recommends using their oven to air roast sheet pan dinners with a protein (like steak, chicken, or seafood), vegetables and spices. After following the oven booklet's recipe for Spicy Chicken, Sweet Potatoes & Broccoli, I was impressed with the result. All of the ingredients (about three pounds in total) came out lightly browned and tender in just 22 minutes and made a tasty sheet pan dinner for four. This technique does seem like a very good use for this appliance.

Baking

The heat inside the oven is evenly distributed for the perfect baking process. Compared to other leading air fryer ovens in the market, it offers 40% even baking.

Air Frying

Sincerely speaking, in contrast to dedicated air fryers, the Ninja Foodi air fryer oven is not the best. This does not mean it's poor but it qualifies as an average air fryer.

Some foods come out unevenly fried and without the full crispy results provided by power air fryer.

Toasting

When it comes to toasting, the Ninja Foodi oven does a great job.It has the capability to accommodate 9 slices without squishing them.

The results are perfect with great browning and even on all the slices.

Air Broiling

Chicken breasts came out juicy and browned on both sides in just 20 minutes. However, even when cooked well-done, steaks looked gray on the outside and in no way resembled broiled or grilled meat. So, while this oven is fast, it can't consistently deliver the kind of searing you expect from broiling.

Keep Warm

Its warm function can keep food warm for up to 2 hours for serving temperature. Past two hours, the food can get dried up.

Ease of Cleaning

To clean the appliance doesn't require much effort due to the removable tray crumb and easily accessible back panel.

Sheet pan and air fryer basket can be cleaned with a dishwasher.

Instruction Guide

The Ninja Foodi air fryer oven comes with a detailed and easy to read guide. Additional booklet for recipes and cooking charts is provided to make functions like air frying and dehydration understandable.

Warranty

Ninja provides a 1-year limited warranty for the air fryer and a 60-day money-back guarantee. It would be better if the warranty is longer.

BREAKFASTS RECIPES

Air Fryer Bacon and Egg Breakfast Biscuit Bombs

Prep/Cook Time: 50 min, Servings 8

Ingredients

Biscuit Bombs
- 4 slices bacon, cut into 1/2-inch pieces
- 1 tablespoon butter
- 2 eggs, beaten
- 1/4 teaspoon pepper
- 1 can (10.2 oz) Pillsbury™ Grands!™ Southern Homestyle refrigerated Buttermilk biscuits (5 biscuits)
- 2 oz sharp cheddar cheese, cut into ten 3/4-inch cubes

Egg Wash
- 1 egg
- 1 tablespoon water

Instructions

- Cut two 8-inch rounds of cooking parchment paper. Place one round in bottom of air fryer basket. Spray with cooking spray.
- In 10-inch nonstick skillet, cook bacon over medium-high heat until crisp. Remove from pan; place on paper towel. Carefully wipe skillet with paper towel. Add butter to skillet; melt over medium heat. Add 2 beaten eggs and pepper to skillet; cook until eggs are thickened but still moist, stirring frequently. Remove from heat; stir in bacon. Cool 5 minutes.
- Meanwhile, separate dough into 5 biscuits; separate each biscuit into 2 layers. Press each into 4-inch round. Spoon 1 heaping tablespoonful egg mixture onto center of each round. Top with one piece of the cheese. Gently fold edges up and over filling; pinch to seal. In small bowl, beat remaining egg and water. Brush biscuits on all sides with egg wash.
- Place 5 of the biscuit bombs, seam sides down, on parchment in air fryer basket. Spray both sides of second parchment round with cooking spray. Top biscuit bombs in basket with second parchment round, then top with remaining 5 biscuit bombs.
- Set to 325°F; cook 8 minutes. Remove top parchment round; using tongs, carefully turn biscuits, and place in basket in single layer. Cook 4 to 6 minutes longer or until cooked through (at least 165°F).

Nutrition Info

Calories 200, Calories from Fat 100, Total Fat 12g, Saturated Fat 6g, Trans Fat 0g, Cholesterol 85mg

Ninja Foodi hashbrown casserole

Prep/Cook Time: 35 minutes, Servings: 12

Ingredients

- 6 eggs
- 48 oz bag frozen hashbrowns
- 1/4 cup milk
- 1 large onion
- 3 tbs olive oil
- 1 pound Ham
- 1/2 cup cheddar cheese

Instructions

- Turn your Foodi on Saute
- Add olive oil and chopped onion cook on saute till translucent
- Add in frozen hashbrowns. Turn on Air Crips 350 for 15 minutes Flipping half way between
- Mix together eggs and milk
- Pour over your golden hashbrowns and add your breakfast meat
- Add your meat to the top
- Place Foodi on aircrisp 350 for 10 minutes or until top is golden brown and eggs are done.
- Top with Cheddar cheese and close lid till cheese melts about 1 minute

Nutrition Info

Calories: 682 Total Fat: 43g Saturated Fat: 8g Trans Fat: 0g Cholesterol: 184mg Sodium: 1625mg Carbohydrates: 52g Fiber: 5g Sugar: 2g Protein: 24g

Easy Air Fried Chicken Omelets

Prep/Cook Time 23 mins, Servings: 2

Ingredients

- 4 eggs
- 1/2 cup Tyson Grilled & Ready Fully Cooked Oven Roasted Diced Chicken Breast ,divided
- 2 tbsp shredded cheese ,divided
- 1/2 tsp salt ,divided
- 1/4 tsp pepper ,divided
- 1/4 tsp granulated garlic ,divided
- 1/4 tsp onion powder ,divided

Instructions

- Spray 2 ramekins with olive oil.
- Crack two eggs into each ramekin.
- Add cheese and seasonings.
- Whisk to combine.
- Sprinkle in 1/4 cup diced chicken in each cup.
- Bake in the air fryer at 330 degrees Fahrenheit for 14-18 minutes or until fully cooked and no longer runny.

Nutrition Info

Calories: 200kcal, Carbohydrates: 7g, Protein: 15g, Fat: 12g, Saturated Fat: 9.4g

Air Fryer Cinnamon Rolls

Prep/Cook Time 20 minutes, Servings 10

Ingredients

- 1 roll crescent rolls refrigerated
- 1/3 c brown sugar
- 1/3 c butter melted
- 1/4 c raisins
- 1/3 c nuts chopped, pecans or walnuts
- 2 tbsp maple syrup
- 2 tbsp sugar
- 1 tbsp cinnamon

Instructions

- Whisk together your melted butter, brown sugar and maple syrup.
- Put a trivet inside your air fryer/Ninja Foodi and an 8" springform (or other style) pan that's been sprayed with non stick spray on top.
- Pour your brown sugar mixture inside your pan. Sprinkle your nuts and raisins (can add dried cranberries too) into the pan too.
- Open your package of refrigerated crescent rolls but DO NOT unroll the crescent roll roll as you normally would. Instead put it on a cutting board and cut it in half (use a non serrated knife so it doesn't smush down when slicing).
- Then cut those pieces in half again, and again until you get 8 equal pieces.
- Mix your cinnamon and sugar in a bowl and dip the bottom and top of each cut crescent roll piece in it. Then put each one into your pan on top of your brown sugar mixture with the sugar mixture facing up.
- Close your air fryer lid (one attached on the Ninja Foodi) and set to air crisp, 345 degrees, for 5 minutes.
- Open lid and flip each crescent roll piece upside down.
- Turn air fryer on again, press air crisp, 345 degrees for 4 more minutes (5 if you want them crispier on top).
- Immediately remove pan, place cooked sticky buns on a plate and spoon mixture at the bottom of the pan on top of your rolls. Enjoy!!

Nutrition Info

Calories 143 Calories from Fat 72, Fat 8g, Saturated Fat 4g, Cholesterol 16mg, Sodium 58mg, Potassium 77mg, Carbohydrates 17g, Fiber 1g, Sugar 11g, Protein 1g

Air Fryer Donut Recipe

Prep/Cook Time 16 minutes, Servings 6

Ingredients
- 1 roll refrigerated cinnamon rolls not Grands, cut in half and rolled into balls
- 2 tbsp butter melted
- 1/4 c cinnamon
- 1/2 c sugar

Instructions
- Preheat air fryer to 390 degrees. Cut refrigerated cinnamon rolls in half and roll each one into a tight ball.
- Melt butter in a small bowl. Pour cinnamon and sugar into a pint size baggie and shake to mix well.
- Dip each rolled cinnamon roll into the butter so it is coated, then put into the baggie and shake so the outside is coated with cinnamon and sugar.
- Spray air fryer basket with non stick spray and put coated pieced inside basket with room in between them (they will spread a bit). I put 8 pieces in at a time = half the container.
- Close the lid and continue to air fry at 390 degrees for a total of 5-6 minutes, flipping them after minute 3. Check at minute 5 to see if yours are done through, if not use the last minute.
- Put remaining sugar and cinnamon into a new baggie (the other one will be a bit wet). Take each one out one at a time and shake in new baggie to recoat with more sugar and cinnamon.
- Drizzle or dip each one in frosting that came in your cinnamon roll container and enjoy.

Nutrition Info
Calories 312 Calories from Fat 117, Fat 13g, Saturated Fat 6g, Cholesterol 10mg, Sodium 474mg, Carbohydrates 47g, Fiber 1g, Sugar 30g, Protein 3g

Air Fryer Hard Boiled Eggs

Prep/Cook Time 19 minutes, Servings 6

Ingredients

- 6 eggs

Instructions

- Place egg into air fryer, not overlapping.
- ** For best results allow eggs to sit on counter for at least 10 minutes vs. straight out of the very cold fridge.
- Turn machine on, close lid, and set to 270 degrees for: 10 minutes for runny yolks, 14 minutes for yellow but soft yolks (I will say these are perfect), 15 minutes for yolks that are hard but not overcooked so they turn gray
- Remove immediately and put into a bowl filled with cold water and ice cubes.
- Once cooled remove shells and enjoy.

Nutrition Info

Calories 62 Calories from Fat 36, Fat 4g, Saturated Fat 1g, Cholesterol 163mg, Sodium 62mg, Potassium 60mg, Protein 5g

Easy Air Fried Chicken Omelets

Prep/Cook Time 23 mins, Servings: 2

Ingredients

- 4 eggs
- 1/2 cup Tyson® Grilled & Ready® Fully Cooked Oven Roasted Diced Chicken Breast ,divided
- 2 tbsp shredded cheese ,divided
- 1/2 tsp salt ,divided
- 1/4 tsp pepper ,divided
- 1/4 tsp granulated garlic ,divided
- 1/4 tsp onion powder ,divided

Instructions

- Spray 2 ramekins with olive oil.
- Crack two eggs into each ramekin.
- Add cheese and seasonings.
- Whisk to combine.
- Sprinkle in 1/4 cup diced chicken in each cup.
- Bake in the air fryer at 330 degrees Fahrenheit for 14-18 minutes or until fully cooked and no longer runny.

Nutrition Info

Calories: 282, Total Fat: 17g, Saturated Fat: 11g, Trans Fat: 1g Unsaturated Fat: 2g

Air Fryer Breakfast Potatoes

Prep/Cook Time 35 minutes, Servings 6

Ingredients

- 3 large potatoes russet
- 1 onion yellow, diced
- 1 green pepper diced
- 2 tsp salt
- 1/2 tsp pepper
- 2 tbsp olive oil
- 1 c cheese shredded, optional

Instructions

- In a mixing bowl add diced potatoes (with skins on), onions, green peppers and seasonings. Drizzle with olive oil and stir so everything is coated.
- Preheat air fryer for 5 minutes at 400 degrees.
- Pour mixture into air fryer basket and cook for 15-20 minutes shaking every 5 minutes. Take out once potatoes are tender with a fork and browned as much as you'd like.
- If you want to add cheese you can sprinkle it on the last 3-5 minutes to melt, or dump potatoes when done in a dish, sprinkle cheese on top and microwave for about 2 minutes until it is melted.

Nutrition Info

Calories 236 Calories from Fat 99, Fat 11g, Saturated Fat 5g, Cholesterol 20mg, Sodium 912mg, Potassium 842mg, Carbohydrates 26g, Fiber 5g, Sugar 1g, Protein 10g

Homemade Chicken Enchiladas

Prep/Cook Time 40 mins, Servings: 6

Ingredients

- 12 corn tortillas
- 1½ cups Mexican Shredded Chicken
- 2 cups Enchilada Sauce store-bought or homemade
- 1½ cups Mexican Shredded Cheese

Instructions

- Spritz 6 corn tortillas with oil of your choice and line the basket of the NF Air Fry Oven with the tortillas, overlapping them as little as possible. Air Fry on 425°F/220°C for 3-5 minutes or until lightly brown in areas and pliable. Repeat with remaining 6 corn tortillas.
- Add 2-3 Tbsp of filling to each corn tortilla, roll and place in pairs on non-stick tray.
- Spoon about ⅓ cup of enchilada sauce over the tops of each pair.
- Slide the tray in the oven and bake at 325°F/160°C for 20 minutes. Add about ¼ cup of Mexican Shredded Cheese to the top of each pair and return to the oven. Broil on high for 2-3 minutes or until the cheese is melted and bubbly.
- Top with your favorite toppings and Enjoy!

Nutrition Info

Calories: 331kcal, Carbohydrates: 34g, Protein: 24g, Fat: 11g, Saturated Fat: 5g, Cholesterol: 27mg

Instant Pot / Pressure Cooker Egg Bites

Prep/Cook Time: 40 mins, Servings: 14 egg bites

Ingredients

- 8 large eggs
- 1/4 cup milk
- 1/4 teaspoon salt
- 1/8 teaspoon freshly ground black pepper
- 1/2 cup diced ham or precooked bacon (or both!)
- 1/3 cup shredded cheddar cheese
- 1 green onion, optional

Instructions

- Generously spray two silicone baby food trays with nonstick cooking spray. In a large bowl, whisk the eggs, milk, salt, and pepper until just blended. Evenly divide the meat among silicone cups. Pour the egg mixture over the ham until each cup is about two-thirds full. Sprinkle the cheddar cheese over each egg bite.
- Pour 1 cup water into the pressure cooking pot and place a trivet in the bottom. Use a sling to lower the silicone trays, carefully stacking one on top of the other. Lock the lid in place. Select High Pressure and 11 minutes cook time for firmer egg bites. (Take a minute or two off the cook time if you prefer softer eggs.)
- When the cook time ends, turn off the pressure cooker. Let the pressure release naturally for 5 minutes, then finish with a quick pressure release. When the valve drops, carefully remove the lid and use the sling to remove the trays. Place on a wire rack to cool for 5 minutes, then turn the tray over and gently squeeze to remove the egg bites from the silicone trays.
- Serve egg bites whole or sliced on top of mini croissants or toast.

Nutrition Info

Calories: 72 Total Fat: 5g Saturated Fat: 2g Trans Fat: 0g Unsaturated Fat: 3g Cholesterol: 115mg Sodium: 186mg Carbohydrates: 1g Fiber: 0g Sugar: 0g Protein: 6g

POULTRY RECIPES

Pressure Cooker Mexican Rice

Prep/Cook Time 12 minutes, Servings 6

Ingredients

- 2 c white rice uncooked
- 1 c tomato sauce
- 2 1/4 c chicken broth
- 1 tsp garlic powder
- 1 tsp onion powder
- 1/4 tsp ground cumin
- 1/2 tsp salt
- 1/4 tsp pepper
- 1/2 onion diced, optional

Instructions

- Add all ingredients other than your onions and rice and stir. Add onions and stir. Then sprinkle uncooked rice on the top and gently submerge into the liquid. Do not stir or you may receive the burn message.
- Close the pressure cooker lid and set the valve to sealing, then select the pressure cook setting to high for 7 minutes.
- Allow to naturally release steam for 10 minutes when done, then release pressure valve and lift lid.
- Use a fork to fluff rice, stir and serve. Turn pot off. Best if served immediately.

Nutrition Info

Calories 247 Calories from Fat 9, Fat 1g, Saturated Fat 1g, Sodium 735mg, Potassium 296mg, Carbohydrates 54g, Fiber 2g, Sugar 2g, Protein 6g

Ninja Foodi Chicken Breast

Prep/Cook Time 21 minutes, Servings 4

Ingredients
- 3 chicken breasts boneless, skinless preferred
- 1/2 c water
- 3/4 c barbecue sauce
- 1 tsp garlic powder
- 1/2 tsp salt

Instructions
- In a bowl mix together bbq sauce, garlic powder and salt.
- In a separate bowl add 1/2 cup of this bbq sauce mixture + your water and whisk together. Pour this into the bottom of your Foodi pot.
- Lower down a trivet (the metal one your pot came with works perfect)
- Lay chicken breasts on rack and brush on remaining bbq sauce in your bowl on to meat.
- Close lid and steam valve and set to pressure cook high for 6 minutes. Allow to naturally release pressure when done for 3 minutes. (timing will vary depending on how thick your breasts are, always check temp when done to ensure it's done in the middle)
- Lift off pressure cooker lid and set aside.
- Lift out rack with chicken, set aside, and pour out liquid at the bottom of your pot.
- Transfer meat into your air fryer basket and lower into your pot. (you can brush on more bbq sauce now if you want it really layered on)
- Take note: if you follow the next steps to get a bit of crisp on the outside it will dry your chicken out more than if you ate it without the air crisp function. Close air crisp lid and cook at 400 degrees for 4 minutes or until internal temp when removed is 160 degrees.

Nutrition Info
Calories 288 Calories from Fat 45, Fat 5g, Saturated Fat 1g, Cholesterol 108mg, Sodium 1040mg, Potassium 761mg, Carbohydrates 22g, Fiber 1g, Sugar 18g, Protein 37g

Pressure Cooker Chicken and Rice

Prep/Cook Time 20 minutes, Servings 4

Ingredients

- 1 lb chicken breasts cut into cubes, boneless, skinless
- 1 can cream of chicken soup
- 1 c mixed vegetables frozen
- 1 c white rice not instant, we use long grain white rice
- 1 tsp garlic salt
- 1/2 onions diced
- pinch pepper
- 2 c chicken broth could use water
- 1/2 c cheese cheddar, shredded
- 2 tbsp olive oil

Instructions

- Put cubed chicken pieces and diced onions into Instant Pot with olive oil and set to saute, cook until chicken is cooked on the outside (will continue to cook in next step so outside just needs to be cooked/white in color). Turn pot off!
- Sprinkle with seasonings. Add cream of chicken soup, frozen vegetables, and broth into your pressure cooker. Stir together WELL until clumps of cream of chicken are smoothed out.
- Sprinkle rice on top and DO NOT Stir!!
- Put lid on Instant Pot, close steam valve and set to manual, high pressure for 9 minutes.
- Allow to naturally release for 3 minutes when done, let out rest of steam, and carefully lift lid. Add cheese now and stir until melted or serve topped with cheese.

Nutrition Info

Calories 528 Calories from Fat 171, Fat 19g, Saturated Fat 6g, Cholesterol 93mg, Sodium 1209mg, Potassium 743mg, Carbohydrates 51g, Fiber 2g, Sugar 1g, Protein 35g

Ninja Foodi Chicken Tenders

Prep/Cook Time 27 minutes, Servings 4

Ingredients

- 1 lb chicken tenders 8 pcs. came in our package
- 1/2 c bread crumbs Italian style is best
- 1 egg whisked
- 2 tbsp olive oil
- 8 slices bacon optional

Instructions

- Whip your egg in a bowl. In a different bowl combine your bread crumbs with your olive oil. Preheat your air fryer to 350 for 10 minutes while you're preparing your chicken.
- Dip each chicken tender into the egg on both sides letting excess egg drip off before putting it into the bread crumb bowl. Flip over so whole piece of chicken is covered in wet bread crumb mixture.
- If not adding bacon, place these coated pieces into your air fryer basket.
- If wrapping with bacon, cut 8 slices of bacon in half and lay 2 of your half pieces down next to one another horizontally.
- Place your coated chicken tender in the middle. Use 2 toothpicks to secure ends of bacon pieces on to chicken. Insert at an angle so they are somewhat flat so when you put them into the basket they lay relatively flat.
- Place chicken wrapped pieces into air fryer basket with toothpick sides down.
- Once all pieces are in basket and aren't overlapping (we did 2 batches so they didn't) close lid and select air crisp for 12 minutes if there's no bacon, or 14 minutes if you wrapped with bacon.
- Flip chicken pieces halfway through your cook cycle. If you want them really crisp spray oil on them for the last 2 minutes. Remove and enjoy!

Nutrition Info

Calories 443 Calories from Fat 261, Fat 29g, Saturated Fat 7g, Cholesterol 142mg, Sodium 537mg, Potassium 548mg, Carbohydrates 10g, Protein 32g

Instant Pot Shredded Chicken

Prep/Cook Time 15 minutes, Servings 5

Ingredients

- 1 jar barbecue sauce 20 oz. or so, not honey style or one with a lot of sugar in it
- 1 c chunk pineapple
- 3 chicken breasts cut in half or thirds, boneless / skinless, can dice for shorter cook time
- 1 bag flour tortillas pkg. small
- 3/4 c water or use chicken broth
- avocado sliced, optional
- 1 c pineapple juice from the can you're using
- 1 onion sliced, optional
- 1 tbsp soy sauce optional
- 1 c cheese

Instructions

- Empty 1/2 jar of barbecue sauce on bottom of Instant Pot. (do not use honey variety as that will burn)
- Put chicken breasts on top of your sauce. Make sure they are cut in half or thirds so they cook through. You can dice into bite size pcs. too for a shorter cook time. Then squeeze the other half of jar on top of the chicken.
- Pour 3/4 c water or broth inside your bbq sauce jar. Put lid on and shake, pour this on top of chicken followed by chunks of pineapple (and sliced onion + soy sauce if you choose to add that). Gently stir so chicken is well coated. If you dice the chicken into bite size pieces, set to high for 5 min.
- Close Instant Pot and make sure steam valve is closed. Set to poultry setting, high for 15 minutes (automatically sets to this time when you hit the poultry function, very thick breasts may take longer to become very tender to shred).
- When it beeps do a quick release, and then lift lid.
- Use 2 forks to shred chicken right in the pot. Add some to small tortillas to make soft tacos with some cheese and avocado, or leave chicken whole and serve on top of rice.

Nutrition Info

Calories 170 Calories from Fat 63, Fat 7g, Saturated Fat 4g, Cholesterol 20mg, Sodium 165mg, Potassium 167mg, Carbohydrates 20g, Fiber 1g, Sugar 16g, Protein 6g

Frozen Chicken Breast in Air Fryer

Prep/Cook Time 20 minutes, Servings 2

Ingredients

- 2 large chicken breasts frozen, boneless skinless is what was used
- 1/2 tsp salt
- 1/4 tsp pepper
- 1/4 tsp garlic powder
- 1/4 tsp parsley flakes

Instructions

- Put frozen chicken breasts in your air fryer basket. Sprinkle ingredients on top evenly between the two of them.
- Close and cook at 360 degrees for 15 minutes. Remove and check to ensure they are done (some are thicker than others so may need additional time). Allow to sit for 5 minutes to maintain juices before slicing them.

Nutrition Info

Calories 260 Calories from Fat 54, Fat 6g, Saturated Fat 1g, Cholesterol 145mg, Sodium 844mg, Potassium 836mg, Carbohydrates 1g, Sugar 1g, Protein 48g

Pressure Cooker Chicken Taco Bowls

Prep/Cook Time 27 minutes, Servings 6

Ingredients

- 1 lb chicken boneless, skinless, breasts
- 2 tbsp olive oil
- 1/4 c taco seasoning
- 1/2 tsp salt optional
- 1 c chicken broth
- 1 can corn drained
- 1 can black beans drained
- 1 c rice white, uncooked
- 1 jar salsa 15.5 oz.

Instructions

- Put olive oil in pot and turn pressure cooker to saute function. Place chicken breasts into pot and allow to cook each side for about 2 min. per side so the outsides are no longer pink. Turn pot off. Move chicken to the side and pour in a bit of your broth so you can deglaze your pot. (meaning scrape bits of stuck on chicken off the bottom of your pot)
- Sprinkle taco seasoning on top of breasts. Pour chicken broth on top of that, then add salt if desired, followed by the can of corn. Spread kernels out evenly inside pot.
- Add drained can of beans on top of that, spread out evenly. Sprinkle in uncooked rice evenly inside pot.
- Pour jar of salsa on top of rice so all of it is covered.
- Close pressure cooker lid and steam valve to sealed.
- Set to pressure cook, high, for 12 minutes. Then do a quick release.
- Remove chicken breasts and put on a bowl to shred. Then put back into your pot with other ingredients and stir.
- Serve this in bowls topped with: sour cream avocado, cheese, etc!

Nutrition Info

Calories 373 Calories from Fat 108, Fat 12g, Saturated Fat 2g, Cholesterol 27mg, Sodium 1162mg, Potassium 432mg, Carbohydrates 55g, Fiber 8g, Sugar 5g, Protein 15g

Pressure Cooker Chicken Noodle Casserole

Prep/Cook Time 12 minutes, Servings 6

Ingredients

- 2 c chicken precooked - I used diced rotisserie chicken
- 1 c mixed vegetables we used frozen, could use canned
- 2 c chicken broth
- 1.5 c noodles small, we used farfalle
- 1/4 tsp garlic salt
- 3 tbsp cornstarch
- 1/4 c half and half
- 1/2 c cheese more if desired
- 1 can cream of chicken soup

Instructions

- If using precooked chicken (leftovers or rotisserie are great) make sure it is diced into bite size pieces and put it into your pressure cooker.
- If using fresh chicken (make sure pieces are diced into small bite size pieces) set pot to saute with 1 tbsp olive oil and cook until outsides are no longer pink. Then turn pot off.
- Add mixed vegetables, uncooked noodles, and garlic salt into your pot with your chicken.
- In a bowl whisk together your broth and cream of chicken soup so it is smooth/well combined. Dump this into your Instant Pot and stir all contents together.
- Close your lid and steam valve and set to high pressure for 2 minutes.
- Do a quick release and stir contents.
- Set your pot to saute again.
- In a bowl whisk together half and half and cornstarch until smooth, pour this mixture into your pot once contents are bubbling.
- Stir, will thicken quickly. Stir in cheese and allow to melt. Turn pot off and pour contents into a serving dish so it doesn't continue to cook and noodles get too soft.

Nutrition Info

Calories 272 Calories from Fat 117, Fat 13g, Saturated Fat 5g, Cholesterol 45mg, Sodium 844mg, Potassium 278mg, Carbohydrates 23g, Fiber 1g, Protein 14g

Instant Pot Crack Chicken Casserole

Prep/Cook Time 25 minutes, Servings 6

Ingredients

- 2 lbs chicken thighs boneless skinless, cubed - can use chicken breasts if preferred
- 8 oz cream cheese softened, room temp.
- 3 strips bacon diced
- 3 tbsp olive oil
- 1 packet ranch seasoning dry mix in packet
- 2 c chicken broth
- 5 c egg noodles use measuring cup to measure 5 cups uncooked into pot
- 1/2 c peas frozen, optional
- 1/2 onion diced, optional

Instructions

- Set Instant Pot to saute and add olive oil and bacon.
- Cook for a few minutes until bacon is consistently sizzling and almost done. (add onion now if you want to add it)
- Add cubed chicken thigh pieces and cook until outsides of chicken are no longer pink. Turn Instant Pot off/cancel so it can cool a bit before turning it to high pressure. Scrape remaining bits of meat off bottom of pot.
- Sprinkle ranch seasoning packet on top of bacon and chicken and mix gently.
- Cut softened cream cheese into clumps and put on top of chicken mixture, followed by 1/2 cup of chicken broth.
- Close lid and steam valve and set to high pressure for 5 minutes.
- Do a quick release, stir contents gently allowing cream cheese bits to become creamy and no longer clumped up.
- Add your frozen peas, then 5 measuring cups full of uncooked small egg noodles, and then your remaining 1.5 c. of chicken broth on top of your noodles.
- Gently stir just a bit.
- Close lid and steam valve and set to high pressure for 3 minutes.
- Do a quick release, stir and serve!!
- If you want sauce a bit thicker turn IP to saute again to have liquid bubble for 1-2 minutes and stir gently while bubbling. Allow to sit and the longer it sits the thicker it will get.

Nutrition Info

Calories 707 Calories from Fat 459, Fat 51g, Saturated Fat 16g, Cholesterol 223mg, Sodium 605mg, Potassium 566mg, Carbohydrates 27g, Fiber 1g, Sugar 2g, Protein 33g

Instant Pot Lemon Garlic Chicken

Prep/Cook Time 20 minutes, Servings 4

Ingredients

- 4 chicken thighs bone in, skinless
- 2 tbsp olive oil
- 1/2 onion diced
- 2 tbsp minced garlic
- 1/2 tsp salt adjust to taste when done
- 1/2 tsp pepper adjust to taste when done
- 1/4 c parsley fresh, chopped finely
- 3/4 c chicken broth
- 3 tbsp butter melted
- 1 large lemon juiced, 3 tbsp juice
- 2 tbsp cornstarch + water to whisk and thicken

Instructions

- Set pot to saute and pour in olive oil until hot. Put thighs in pot and brown both sides. Then remove meat.
- Add diced onion, garlic, parsley, salt and pepper. Saute together for about 2 minutes while scraping bits of chicken off bottom of pot to deglaze. Pour in 1/4 c. chicken broth once onions have softened and finish deglazing pot.
- Turn pot off. Add thighs back into pot.
- Pour rest of chicken broth in around chicken. Pour melted butter on chicken as well as lemon juice.
- Close lid and steam valve and set to high pressure for 10 minutes (for medium thighs with bone in).
- Do a quick release and remove thighs, set aside to keep warm.
- Set pot to saute again. In a small bowl whisk together cornstarch and a bit of water until smooth. When liquid in pot bubbles, add this and stir. Allow to thicken for a few minutes and turn pot off.
- Serve thighs with sauce poured on top. Season with more salt and pepper to taste.

Nutrition Info

Calories 417 Calories from Fat 315, Fat 35g, Saturated Fat 11g, Cholesterol 133mg, Sodium 618mg, Potassium 345mg, Carbohydrates 8g, Fiber 1g, Sugar 1g, Protein 19g

DESSERTS RECIPES

Pepperoni Pizza Pasta

Prep/Cook Time 30 minutes, Servings: 8

Ingredients

- 1/4 teaspoon ground black pepper
- 1/4 teaspoon crushed red pepper
- 6 large cloves garlic, minced or pressed
- 1 cup red wine
- 1 lb. Itallian Sausage
- 1 large onion, diced
- 1 teaspoon kosher salt
- 1 box (16 ounces) dry rigatoni pasta
- 4 cups shredded mozzarella cheese, divided
- 1 package (6 ounces) thin-sliced pepperoni
- 1/2 teaspoon dried oregano
- 1/2 teaspoon dried basil
- 1 can (28 ounces) peeled San Marzano tomatoes
- 1 can (28 ounces) San Marzano tomato puree
- 2 cups chicken stock

Instructions

- Select Saute (Sear/Saute MD:Hi on the Foodi). Preheat pot for 5 minutes. Cook sausage until browned and crumbled. Remove to a plate lined with paper towels.
- Add onion and olive oil to the pot. Cook for 2 minutes. Add salt, oregano, basil, black pepper, and crushed red pepper. Continue cooking, stirring occasionally until onions are lightly browned and translucent, about 5 minutes.
- Add browned sausage, garlic. wine, tomatoes, tomato puree, chicken stock, and pasta to the pot and stir to combine. Lock the pressure cooking lid in place.
- Select High Pressure and 6 minute cook time. If necessary, press start to begin.
- When pressure cooking is complete, allow pressure to natural release for 10 minutes. After 10 minutes, quick release remaining pressure. Carefully remove the lid.
- Stir the sauce with a wooden spoon, crushing tomatoes in the process.
- Cover pasta mixture with 3 cups shredded mozzarella. Lay pepperoni slices across mozzarella. Sprinkle remaining mozzarella over pepperoni slices. (If you're not using the Foodi to melt and brown the cheese, transfer pasta to a 9x13 pan before topping with cheese.)
- Foodi: Close crisping lid. Select Air Crisp, set temperature to 400ºF and set time to 5 minutes. Select Start to begin. Oven: Preheat oven to 400ºF and cook until cheese is melted and browned.
- Serve immediately.

Nutrition Info

Calories: 465 Total Fat: 25g Saturated Fat: 10g Trans Fat: 0g Unsaturated Fat: 13g Cholesterol: 79mg Sodium: 1141mg Carbohydrates: 29g Fiber: 3g Sugar: 9g Protein: 26g

Ninja Foodi Kale Chips

Prep/Cook Time 15 minutes, Servings 6

Ingredients

- 1 bunch kale curly kale is best, washed, dried, remove stems
- 2 tbsp olive oil
- 1/4 tsp seasoned salt or 1/2 tsp. dry ranch dressing mix

Instructions

- Wash your kale and set out on countertop on paper towels to completely dry.
- Remove middle stems and cut leaves into large bite size pieces, they will shrink.
- Put pieces into a bowl and drizzle olive oil on, sprinkle on seasoned salt or ranch dressing seasoning.
- Use hands to massage salt and oil on to leaves.
- Put half your prepared bunch into your air fryer basket
- Close your air fryer lid (attached on Ninja Foodi), press air crisp at 390 degrees for 2 minutes.
- Lift lid and flip kale chips on to the other side to crisp evenly.
- Re set air crisp at 390 degrees for another 2 minutes (or set to 4 minutes and flip halfway through). Then remove and do the same for the 2nd half of your batch of prepared kale.
- Kale chips should be crispy on both sides, if you have a bit larger bunch you may need to add another minute at the very end to ensure all pieces are very crispy like chips. Enjoy immediately for best results.

Nutrition Info

Calories 51 Calories from Fat 36, Fat 4g, Sodium 105mg, Potassium 106mg, Carbohydrates 1g

Instant Pot Chili Recipe No Beans

Prep/Cook Time: 20 M, Servings: 4

Ingredients:

- 1 Onion, diced
- 1 Green Pepper, diced
- 1 Tbs Salt
- 1 Tbs Smoked Paprika
- 1/4 tsp Cayenne Pepper
- 2 lbs Grass-fed Ground Beef
- 1 Tbs Minced Garlic
- 1 Tbs Avocado Oil
- 3 Tbs Chili Powder
- 1 Tbs Cumin
- 21 oz Fire Roasted Diced Tomatoes (1.5 cans)
- 2 Tbs Tomato Paste
- 4oz can Green Chilies
- Juice from 1 lime
- 3 Bay Leaves

Instructions:

- Set Ninja Foodi/ instant pot to Saute, medium-high heat and add diced onion, green pepper, and avocado oil and saute for about 2 minutes.
- Add ground beef, salt, smoked paprika, cayenne pepper, chili powder, and cumin. Stir and saute until ground beef is browned
- Drain canned tomatoes and add to the pot along with the green chilies, tomato paste, and lime juice. Stir until well combined.
- Add bay leaves, put the pressure cooker lid on and pressure cook on high for 10 minutes
- Once it finishes cooking let it sit for 5 minutes to relieve the pressure. After 5 minutes flip the vent knob over to vent (careful it will be hot), let all the steam vent out.
- Remove the lid, give it a good stir and serve.
- Serve with your favorite toppings, Low Carb Cheddar Biscuits or Keto "cornbread"

Nutrition Info

Calories 259, Fat (grams) 15.2, Sat. Fat (grams) 5.8, Net carbs 5, Protein (grams) 21.5

Ninja Foodi Asian Sticky Wings

Prep/Cook Time45 mins, Servings: 2

Ingredients

- 2 tsp red chili pepper paste see recipe to make your own or look for Gourmet Garden in your local grocery store
- 1 tsp ginger fresh and grated
- 1 lb Chicken Wings
- 1 tsp sea salt divided
- 1/4 cup honey
- 1/2 cup rice vinegar
- 1 small orange zest and juice

Instructions

- Add 2 cups of water to the inner pot and place the rack in the low position inside the pot. Place wings on a single layer on the rack that came with your Ninja Foodi on the low position. Place the pressure lid on and turn the valve to seal. Set pressure on High and the time for 2 minutes. When the time is up, immediately release the pressure and remove the lid when all the pressure has been released.
- In a bowl, combine rice vinegar, zest & juice from a small orange or tangelo, red pepper paste, freshly grated ginger, 1/2 tsp fine grind sea salt, honey.
- Remove the chicken wings from the rack and place on paper towels. Pat dry until as much moisture has been removed as possible. Salt wings with remaining 1/2 tsp fine grind sea salt.
- Put the Asian sauce in the inner pot of the Ninja Foodi. Place the rack in the low position into the inner pot. Put the dried wings in a single layer on the rack. Set the Tender Crisp function to 390° F. for 30 minutes. Flip the wings every 10 minutes until desired color is reached.
- Dump wings into pot and stir to coat with sauce. Remove from pot and allow to cool slightly before eating. Enjoy!

Optional Toppings

Sprinkle wings with crushed peanuts, chopped cilantro, and / or chopped green onions.

Nutrition Info

Calories: 440kcal, Carbohydrates: 42g, Protein: 23g, Fat: 19g, Saturated Fat: 5g, Cholesterol: 94mg, Sodium: 1256mg, Potassium: 318mg, Fiber: 1g, Sugar: 39g

Spinach & Artichoke Dip- Ninja Foodi Recipe

Prep/Cook Time: 20 minutes, Servings: 8 Servings

Ingredients

- ½ Cup mayonnaise
- ½ Cup chicken broth
- ½ Cup sour cream
- 8 oz. Mozzarella cheese
- 8 oz. Parmesan cheese
- 8 oz. Pepper jack cheese
- 8 oz. Cream Cheese
- 10 oz. frozen spinach- thawed
- 1 Tablespoon minced garlic
- 1 14 oz. Can artichokes drained

Instructions

- Add garlic to Ninja Foodi
- Add chicken broth
- Add mayonnaise
- Add sour cream
- Add spinach
- Add cream cheese
- Add Artichokes
- Stir until combined
- Close pressure cooker lid- move valve to "seal" position
- Cook on high pressure 4 minutes
- Quick release pressure and remove lid
- Stir and add cheese

Tips

- If you love artichokes as much as I do, add a second can of them to this recipe...you won't be disappointed!
- Eat while it's warm. With all of the Cheesy goodness in this recipe, it is much better when it's served warm.
- Serve with Hawaiian bread! The sweetness of the Hawaiian bread pairs well with the creamy salty goodness of the Ninja Foodi Spinach & Artichoke dip. Use shredded Parmesan instead of grated. The grated Parmesan creates a grainy texture where the shredded creates gooey cheesy goodness!

Nutrition Info

Calories: 222kcal, Serving: 1g, Saturated Fat: 6g Trans Fat: 9g

VEGETARIAN RECIPES

Ninja Baked Potato Soup

Prep/Cook Time: 2 hours 20 mins, Servings: 6-8

Ingredients

- 10 to 12 strips bacon, cooked, drained, and crumbled
- 1 1/4 cups shredded mild cheddar cheese
- 1 cup (8 ounces) sour cream
- 2/3 cup butter
- 2/3 cup flour
- 7 cups milk
- 4 large baking potatoes, baked, cooled, peeled and cubed, about 4 cups
- 4 green onions, (including tops) chopped
- 3/4 teaspoon salt
- 1/2 teaspoon pepper
- Celery salt, (optional to be sprinkled on top of each bowl)

Instructions

- Bake potatoes until fork tender. Cut potatoes in halves. Scoop out and set aside. I chop the potatoes with peels. Add as many peels as you would like and discard the remainder.
- Turn Ninja to Stove Top High. Melt butter. Slowly blend in flour with a wire whisk till thoroughly blended. Gradually add milk, whisking constantly. Whisk in salt and pepper, stirring constantly.
- When the milk mixture is very hot; stir in the potatoes. Add green onions and potato peels. Add sour cream & crumpled bacon. Switch to Slow Cook for 2 hours. You may not need to cook it that long, or even turn it to Buffet setting after testing it after an hour. Stir well. Add cheese a little at a time, until it is melted and mixed in. Serve with celery salt sprinkled on top of soup, and crusty French bread.

This baked potato soup recipe Servings 6 to 8.

- Baked Potatoes.
- Use 400-425° - your choice.
- Wrap the potatoes in foil on Oven setting 425° for an hour on the rack.
- or, aluminum foil seasoned & pierced potatoes, double wrapped, and put them in the pot. Going to turn them after 30 minutes to keep from burning, 425°F, 50 minutes - 1 hour! PERFECT!
- Or... place on rack and don't wrap them.
- And now on the Pyramid mat. No turning - 425° about an hour 10 minutes for 5 big potatoes. Not cutting your mat works the best for the potatoes because it will be across the bottom and go up the sides. The potatoes can rest alongside the pot and no turning no scorching. Love it!

Nutrition Info

Calories: 329 kcal, Saturated Fat: 5g Trans Fat: 7g

Instant Pot Cabbage Roll Soup

Prep/Cook Time: 20 minutes, Servings: 4

Ingredients

- 5 cups cabbage chopped
- 1 28 ounce can diced tomatoes
- 1 10 oz can tomato soup
- 1 TBSP Olive Oil
- 1 large onion diced
- 3 cloves garlic minced
- 1 lb lean ground beef (FOR FREEZER MEAL: 1 bag cooked ground beef)
- 2/3 cup uncooked long grain rice
- 5 cups beef broth
- 1 1/2 cups V8 or other vegetable juice
- 1 teaspoon paprika
- 1 teaspoon thyme
- 1 tablespoon Worcestershire sauce
- 1 lb cooked and drained bacon for garnish

Instructions

- Turn Instant Pot on to SAUTE and add olive oil.
- Add the onion and garlic, and cook 2-3 minutes.
- Add ground beef, brown the meat.
- Once browned, hit CANCEL.
- Carefully pour off any excess grease.
- Add remaining ingredients. Stir ingredients to combine.
- Close the pressure cooking lid, make sure it's in the sealing position and turn toggle to seal.
- Press Pressure (it should automatically set to HIGH pressure, change to low pressure). Set time to 12 minutes, low pressure. Hit START. When finished do a quick release.
- Open the pot and stir everything together. Season with salt and pepper, to taste.
- Garish with cooked bacon.

Nutrition Info

Calories: 424 Total Fat: 23g Saturated Fat: 8g Trans Fat: 0g Unsaturated Fat: 14g Cholesterol: 85mg Sodium: 1529mg Carbohydrates: 20g Fiber: 4g Sugar: 9g Protein: 33g

Pressure Cooker Lentil Soup

Prep/Cook Time: 35mins, Servings: 4

Ingredients

- 2 celery ribs, chopped
- 1 teaspoon ground cumin
- 8 cups vegetable broth
- 1/2 large onion, chopped
- 4 garlic cloves, minced
- 5 ounces fresh spinach (optional)
- salt and pepper
- 2 tablespoons olive oil
- 2 carrots, chopped
- 1 cup dry lentils, rinsed and picked
- 2 bay leaves

Instructions

- In your pressure cooker, sweat the onions and garlic in the olive oil until the onions are translucent.
- Add the carrots and celery and saute for a minute or two.
- Add the ground cumin and stir well.
- Add the vegetable broth, lentils, and bay leaves, close the pressure cooker, and bring up to pressure.
- Cook for 20 minutes.
- Open the pressure cooker via the quick release method (see your cooker's owner's manual!) or let the pressure come down on its own.
- Remove the bay leaves.
- If desired, stir in the spinach, and stir until it wilts. (Additional heat is not necessary.).
- Season with salt and fresh ground pepper to taste.

Nutrition Info

Calories: 403 kcal, Sodium: 190mg Carbohydrates: 16g Fiber: 9g Sugar: 7.3g Protein: 4g

Instant Pot Vegetable Curry

Prep/Cook Time: 20 minutes, Servings: 4

Ingredients

- 1 white onion; diced
- 1/2 cup vegetable broth
- 10 cherry tomatoes; sliced in havles
- 2 zucchini; peeled and diced
- 2 tablespoons yellow curry powder
- 6 carrots; diced
- 1 orange bell pepper; diced
- 1/2 teaspoon salt
- 1/2 teaspoon cracked black pepper

Instructions

- Place all ingredients except tomatoes into the instant pot/pressure cooker. Set to high pressure for 5 minutes. Release pressure when complete.
- Stir well. Top with salt, pepper, and tomatoes. Serve over steamed jasmine rice.

Nutrition Info

Calories: 62 Sodium: 325mg Carbohydrates: 13g Fiber: 3g Sugar: 7g Protein: 2g

Pressure Cooker Vegetable Soup

Prep/Cook Time 35 mins, Servings: 10

Ingredients

- 14.5 ounces fire roasted tomatoes
- 2 tsp sea salt
- 1 tsp onion powder
- 1 lb carrots sliced
- 2 celery
- 1/2 tsp black pepper
- 1 cup 15 bean mix dry
- 4 cups water
- 1/2 Tbsp minors vegetable base
- 1 cup onion diced
- 1 tsp basil dried leaves
- 1 tsp thyme dried leaves
- 1 tsp garlic powder
- 12 ounces corn frozen
- 12 ounces peas frozen
- 12 ounces green beans frozen

Instructions

- Peel and slice carrots into 1/4" slices. Dice onion and celery to 1/2-1" dice. Rinse the beans
- Combine all ingredients into the inner pot of the Ninja Foodi and stir. Put on the pressure lid and make sure the valve is to seal. Pressure cook on high for 30 minutes.
- When the 30 minutes is up, allow to natural release for 3-6 minutes and then manually release the remaining pressure.
- Serve and Enjoy!

Nutrition Info

Calories: 175kcal, Carbohydrates: 35g, Protein: 9g, Sodium: 512mg, Potassium: 421mg, Fiber: 5g

FISH AND SEAFOOD RECIPES

Pressure Cooker Salmon

Prep/Cook Time 9 minutes, Servings 2

Ingredients

- 1 sprig dill fresh
- 1 pinch salt optional
- 3/4 lb salmon filet
- 1/2 lemon juiced
- 1 tbsp butter we used I Can't Believe It's Not Butter
- 1 pinch garlic salt

Instructions

- Pour 1.5 c water into your pressure cooker and lower down a trivet.
- Make a "boat" using foil so butter doesn't drip down into your inner pot. Put your piece of salmon on your foil "boat" skin side down.
- Put a slice of lemon (optional) and tbsp. of I Can't Believe It's Not Butter on the top of your salmon filet. (you can alternatively squeeze the lemon on at the end, if you put lemon slice on now the salmon will not be cooked through as much under the lemon itself - personal preference, I prefer a squeeze of lemon after it is done)
- Sprinkle fresh pcs. of dill (or dried) on top as well as a pinch of salt, garlic salt, and pepper.
- Close lid and steam valve and set to high pressure for 4 minutes (for 3/4 lb., 3 min. for smaller pieces or if you like it under done and quite pink). Do a quick release.
- Lift out fish, use a spatula to remove from foil boat or trivet and enjoy!

Nutrition Info

Calories 293 Calories from Fat 144, Fat 16g, Saturated Fat 5g, Cholesterol 108mg, Sodium 145mg, Potassium 833mg, Protein 33g

Swordfish and Aloha Rice and Vegetables

Prep/Cook Time 1 hour 45 minutes, Servings 2

Ingredients

- 1 tablespoon soy sauce (liquid aminos is a suitable substitute)
- 1 tablespoon honey
- 1 tablespoon apple cider vinegar
- 1 teaspoon ground ginger
- 1 cup long grain brown rice uncooked
- 1 cup chicken stock
- 3 cups water
- 1 (8 oz) can crushed pineapple with liquid
- 1/2 cup green bell pepper diced
- 1/2 cup onion diced
- 1 teaspoon garlic powder
- 1/8 teaspoon crushed red pepper
- 3 carrots peeled and cut into 2-inch chunks
- 1 cup broccoli florets
- 2 (3 oz) swordfish steaks
- 1 teaspoon sesame seeds
- sea salt and freshly ground black pepper to taste

Instructions

- Rinse the brown rice in 2-3 changes of water using a strainer.
- Place the rice, chicken stock and 3 cups water in the Ninja Cooking System and set the dial to STOVE TOP HIGH. Bring to a boil (this takes approximately 10 minutes), then turn the dial to STOVE TOP MEDIUM. Place the lid on the cooker and cook for 20 minutes.
- In the meantime, combine the pineapple, green bell pepper, onion, soy sauce, honey, vinegar, ginger, garlic powder and crushed red pepper in a bowl. Stir to combine. You may also use this time to prep the carrots and broccoli if necessary.
- After the rice has cooked initially for 20 minutes, open the cooker. Pour in the pineapple mixture and stir to combine with rice. Replace the lid, and cook another 15 minutes.
- Open the cooker. Insert the roasting rack. Place the carrots and swordfish steaks on top of the rack. Sprinkle sesame seeds, salt and pepper over vegetables and fish. Replace the lid and allow to cook covered for 10 minutes.
- Open the cooker. Add broccoli and cook another 5 minutes.
- Turn off the cooker. Remove the rack with the swordfish and vegetables. Scoop rice onto a plate and serve topped with swordfish and vegetables.

Nutrition Info

Calories: 351 Saturated Fat: 10g Cholesterol: 45mg Sodium: 758mg Carbohydrates: 35g Fiber: 2g Sugar: 2g Protein: 10g

Ninja Foodi Shrimp Boil Recipe

Prep/Cook Time 25 minutes, Servings 6 people

Ingredients

- 4 cups water
- 1 1/2 Tbsp Zataran's shrimp boil liquid
- 3 tsp Old Bay seasoning divided
- 1 lb red potatoes cut in half
- 4 ears fresh corn snapped in half
- 12 oz cajun style andouille sausage cut into 2 inch pieces
- 1 lb fresh shrimp peeled and deveined
- 1 lb fresh mussels
- fresh chopped parsley optional
- Lemon slices optional

Garlic Butter for Dipping

- 1/2 cup butter melted
- 1/2 tsp garlic powder

Instructions

- Add red potatoes, corn, sausage, water, shrimp boil liquid, and 2 tsp old bay to the Ninja Foodi insert and stir. Cover and cook on high pressure for 4 minutes. Once timer is complete, do a quick release and open lid once all pressure is released.
- Add shrimp and mussels and 1 tsp of old bay. Stir. Cover and cook on high pressure for 1 minute. Once timer goes off, allow to natural release for 2 minutes, then quick release remaining pressure.
- Combine butter and garlic powder in a separate bowl and use as a dipping sauce.
- Sprinkle with parsley and serve with lemon on the side. Enjoy

Nutrition Info

Calories: 1844 Total Fat: 112g Saturated Fat: 40g Trans Fat: 1g Unsaturated Fat: 66g Cholesterol: 433mg Sodium: 2593mg Carbohydrates: 85g

Steamed King Crab Legs with Garlic Butter and Lemon

Prep/Cook Time 10 mins, Servings: 2 -4

Ingredients

- 1 stick of salted butter melted
- 1 large clove of garlic minced
- 2 lbs king crab legs
- Lemon wedges

Instructions

- Melt the butter and minced garlic together in a small pan and keep warm on its lowest setting.
- Set a steamer tray inside a large pot and pour enough water inside to steam the crab. You are only reheating the crab, so you will only need a couple inches of water.
- Add a few cloves of garlic to the water, if desired.
- Bring water to a boil before laying the crab legs on the steamer. Cover the pot and steam for 5 minutes.
- Remove the crab legs and serve with melted garlic butter and lemon wedges. Enjoy!!!

Nutrition Info

Calories: 170 Total Fat: 9g Saturated Fat: 4g Trans Fat: 1g Unsaturated Fat: 5g Cholesterol: 22mg Sodium: 130mg Carbohydrates: 6g

Ninja Foodi Bang Bang Shrimp

Prep/Cook Time 35 mins, Servings: 4 Servings

Ingredients

- ½ cup All purpose flour
- 2 large Eggs
- 1 cup Fine breadcrumbs Can substitute Planko breadcrumbs if desired
- 2 tbsp Grapeseed oil Can substitute olive oil
- 1 tsp Garlic powder
- ½ tsp Kosher salt
- ½ tsp Black pepper, ground
- 1 lb Uncooked large shrimp If frozen they should be thawed first
- ⅓ cup Mayonnaise
- ⅓ cup Sweet and spicy Thai chili sauce
- 1 tbsp Sriracha sauce
- 1 tbsp Lime juice
- 2 tsp Honey Add more to taste and get to the right heat level.
- Kosher salt to taste

Instructions

- Usign three shallow bowls set up dipping station. In the first bowl add the flour, in the second whisk the eggs. In the third coma one the breadcrumbs, Blair powder, oil, salt and pepper.
- Coat shrimp in flour shaking off excess. Dip in egg. Roll in the breadcrumb mixture.
- Preheat the Foodi to 400° and set time for 5 minutes.
- Once preheated and 5 minutes is complete, open lid and add shrimp As a single layer to the basket. If you have the Cook and Crisp insert in Foodi that allows for a secod layer go ahead and use. Set Air Crisp temperature to 400° for 10 minutes, 12 minutes if using the Cookand Crisp insert. Repeat with other batches as needed.
- Breaded shrimp
- While shrimp is cooking make the sauce. Whisk together the mayonoise, sweetand spicy Thai chili sauce, sriracha sauce, lime juice and honey. Make sure they are well combined and then add salt to taste. I did not add any additional salt. I did separate some sauce to a separate bowl and added more honey.
- Bang Bang sauce
- When shrimp are complete drizzle some sauce over shrimp and the serve the remaining sauce for dipping.

Nutrition Info

Calories: 322kcal, Carbohydrates: 45g, Protein: 30g, Fat: 19g, Saturated Fat: 4g, Cholesterol: 146mg, Sodium: 642mg

Steamed Fish Fillet

Prep/Cook time: 20 minutes, Servings: 4

Ingredients:
- 1 clove of garlic, crushed
- a large pinch of fresh thyme
- 4 white fish fillets
- ½ kg cherry tomatoes, sliced
- 1 cup olives
- olive oil
- salt and pepper, to taste

Instructions:
- Heat the pressure cooker and add a cup of water.
- Put the fish fillets in a single layer in the steaming basket fitted for the pressure cooker.
- Place the sliced cherry tomatoes and olives on top of the fillets. Add the crushed garlic, a few sprigs of fresh thyme, a dash of olive oil, and a little salt.
- Put the steaming basket inside the pressure cooker. Seal the lid of the cooker properly.
- Once it reaches pressure, reduce heat. Cook the fillets for 7-10 minutes on low pressure (or 3-5 minutes on high pressure).
- When finished, release pressure through the normal release method.
- Serve the fillets in separate bowls, sprinkled with the remaining thyme, pepper, and little amount of olive oil.

Nutrition Info
Calories: 30, Total Fat: 1g, Protein: 1g

Air Fryer Catfish

Prep/Cook Time: 25 minutes, Servings: 4

Ingredients

- 4 Catfish Fillets or Catfish Nuggets
- 1/2 Cup Gluten Free Fish Fry
- Olive Oil Cooking Spray

Instructions

- Coat each catfish fillet or nugget with an even coat of fish fry.
- Place in the air fryer and spray the olive oil spray on one side of the catfish.
- Cook at 390* for 10 minutes.
- Carefully flip the catfish, coat with spray, and cook for an additional 10 minutes.
- Serve.

Nutrition Info

Calories: 212kcal, Carbohydrates: 9g, Protein: 35g, Fat: 3g, Saturated Fat: 1g, Cholesterol: 85mg, Sodium: 91mg

Air Fryer Shrimp Fajitas {Ninja Foodi}

Prep/Cook Time: 32 minutes, Servings: 12

Ingredients

- 1/2 Cup Sweet Onion, Diced
- 1 Pound Medium Shrimp, Tail-Off (Cooked, Frozen Shrimp)
- 1 Red Bell Pepper, Diced
- 1 Green Bell Pepper, Diced
- 2 Tbsp of Gluten-Free Fajita or Taco Seasoning
- Olive Oil Spray
- White Corn Tortillas or Flour Tortillas

Instructions

- Spray the air fryer basket with olive oil spray or line with foil.
- If the shrimp is frozen with ice on it, run cold water over it to get the ice off.
- Add the shrimp, peppers, onion, and seasoning to the basket.
- Add a coat of olive oil spray.
- Mix it all together.
- Cook at 390 degrees for 12 minutes using the air fryer or air crisp function of the Ninja Foodi.
- Open the lid and spray it again and mix it together.
- Cook an additional 10 minutes.
- Serve on warm tortillas.
- This recipe uses cooked, frozen shrimp, it can be made with uncooked shrimp too but may need a few additional minutes of cook time.

Nutrition Info

Calories: 86, Total Fat: 2g, Saturated Fat: 1g, Trans Fat: 0g, Unsaturated Fat: 2g, Cholesterol: 81mg, Sodium: 420mg, Carbohydrates: 6g, Fiber: 1g, Sugar: 1g, Protein: 10g

Ninja Foodi Lobster Tails

Prep/Cook Time 25 minutes, Servings: 4

Ingredients

- 1 tablespoon butter
- pinch of garlic powder
- 2 tablespoons butter, melted
- 2 lobster tails (mine were about 1/2 lb./tail)
- ½ teaspoon salt
- ½ teaspoon pepper
- 1 cup water
- 1 teaspoon paprika
- Melted butter, for dipping (optional)

Instructions

- With a sharp, clean kitchen shears, cut the shell of the lobster tail right down the middle.
- With both hands, pry the shell apart, loosening the meat of the lobster from the bottom, sides and top of the shell (keeping the end of the tail in tact).
- Once the meat is loosened, carefully pull the meat through the top of the shell and place it on top of the opened shell.
- Season lobster meat with salt and pepper.
- Add water and one tablespoon of butter to cooking pot.
- Place Foodi rack in lower position in the pot and position lobster tails on rack.
- Put pressure cooking lid on Foodi and make sure pressure release valve is in the SEAL position.
- Select HIGH PRESSURE for 2 minutes. QUICK RELEASE.
- Combine garlic powder and melted butter.
- Brush tails with garlic butter mixture.
- Sprinkle tails with paprika.
- AIR CRISP at 375º Fahrenheit for two minutes, brushing tails again with garlic butter halfway through cook time.
- Remove tails from Foodi and enjoy with melted butter.

Nutrition Info

Calories: 161 Total Fat: 6g Saturated Fat: 2g Trans Fat: 0g Unsaturated Fat: 3g Cholesterol: 124mg Sodium: 229mg Carbohydrates: 20g

Air-Fried Crumbed Fish

Prep/Cook Time 22 m, 4 servings

Ingredients

- 4 flounder fillets
- 1 cup dry bread crumbs
- 1/4 cup vegetable oil
- 1 egg, beaten
- 1 lemon, sliced

Instructions

- Preheat an air fryer to 350 degrees F (180 degrees C).
- Mix bread crumbs and oil together in a bowl. Stir until mixture becomes loose and crumbly.
- Dip fish fillets into the egg; shake off any excess. Dip fillets into the bread crumb mixture; coat evenly and fully.
- Lay coated fillets gently in the preheated air fryer. Cook until fish flakes easily with a fork, about 12 minutes. Garnish with lemon slices.

Nutrition Info

354 calories; 17.7 g fat; 22.5 g carbohydrates; 26.9 g protein; 107 mg cholesterol; 309 mg sodium.

BEEF, PORK, AND LAMB -RECIPES-NEED IMAGE FOR 10 RECIPES

Air Fryer Mini Beef Tacos in the Ninja Foodi

Prep/Cook Time 25 mins, Servings: 10 Mini Tacos

Ingredients

- 8 ounces Queso Quesadilla Cheese, Shredded
- cooking spray
- 1 pound ground beef
- 10 Street Taco Shells
- 1 tablespoon taco seasoning

Instructions

- Cook the ground beef until no longer pink. Mix the seasoning into the meat with a half a cup of water. Cook until water is evaporated.
- Mix half the cheese with the ground beef taco meat. Begin heating up the air fryer on 400°.
- Spoon the meat and cheese combination into the street tacos. Top off with the remaining shredded cheese.
- Spray the air fryer basket with cooking spray. Place the mini tacos in the basket. Spray the tops of the tacos with cooking spray.
- Cook for 10 minutes on 400° or until cheese is melted and the shells are crisp.

Nutrition Info

Calories 279 Calories from Fat 153, Fat 17g, Saturated Fat 8g, Cholesterol 56mg, Sodium 370mg, Potassium 168mg, Carbohydrates 16g, Fiber 1g, Sugar 1g, Protein 16g

Braised Lamb Shanks

Prep/Cook Time: 40mins, Servings: 4-6

Ingredients

- 1 garlic clove, crushed
- 1/4 cup plain flour or 1/4 cup gluten-free flour
- 8 teaspoons olive oil
- 1 onion, chopped
- 3 carrots, peeled and thickly sliced
- 3/4 cup red wine
- 1/4 cup beef stock or 1/4 cup vegetable stock
- 1 tablespoon fresh oregano, chopped or 1 teaspoon dried oregano
- 1 teaspoon lemon rind, finely grated
- 2 tomatoes
- 4 -6 lamb shanks, french trimmed if possible
- salt
- fresh ground black pepper
- 4 teaspoons plain flour (optional for thickening gravy) or 4 teaspoons gluten-free flour (optional for thickening gravy)
- 8 teaspoons cold water (optional for thickening gravy)

Instructions

- Peel the tomatoes, remove the calyx and cut into quarters. If you prefer, you can drop the tomatoes into boiling water for one minute and then refresh in ice cold water- this makes removing the skins easier.
- Toss the shanks in the flour -I do this in a large plastic bag for a no mess cleanup. Shake off any excess flour. Discard excess flour.
- Heat half of the oil in the cooker (no lid) and brown the shanks, two at a time if necessary. Remove and set aside.
- Add the remaining oil and the onion, carrots and garlic. Fry for 5 minutes, stirring occassionally. Add the tomatoes, oregano, lemon rind, wine and stock. Bring to the boil, stirring well, for a few minutes.
- Return the lamb shanks to the cooker and season well with salt and pepper. Spoon some of the sauce and vegetables over the meat.
- Close and lock the lid. Set cooker to High Pressure and cook for 25 minutes.
- Carefully release pressure from the cooker and check the meat is cooked. The meat should be very tender and almost falling off the bone. Cook a furtehr 5 minutes if required (though I haven't had to do this).
- If you would like the gravy a little thicker- add the remaining flour to the cold water and stir until smooth. Simmer gravy and add the flour paste in slowly until the gravy is thicker.
- Serve with mashed potato and a green veg -- or baked tiny tomatoes as we did. The green or red really adds colour to the plated meal.

Nutrition Info

Calories: 500 Total Fat: 30g Saturated Fat: 14g Trans Fat: 1g

Ninja Foodi Bacon Wrapped Tenderloin

Prep/Cook Time 21 mins, Servings: 6 Servings

Ingredients

- 2 lbs Pork tenderloin I purchase from my butcher as two 1 lb tenderloins.
- ½ Lb Bacon
- 1 tsp Salt More or less to taste.
- 1 tsp Pepper More or less to taste.
- 1 cup Water

Instructions

- Season the Pork tenderloin with salt and pepper to taste.
- Wrap tenderloin In bacon. Make sure all bacon ends meet on the same side creating a seam you can lat the pork on.
- Bacon wrapped pork tenderloin
- If making potatoes or rice at the same time Either us pot-in-pot method or cover with aluminum foil to capture the pork drippings.
- Pork with potatoes
- Place the cup of water in the Ninja Foodi. Lay the pork tenderloins in a circular pattern on the rack and placed in the Ninja Foodi. If not making potatoes or rice, then place the rack in the low setting, this will prevent having to flip the rack in a future step.
- Set the Ninja Foodi to Pressure and High for 4 minutes. You will be Air Crisping as well, so do not want to overcook. If you prefer your pork more rare cook for 2-3 minutes.
- Once complete release the pressure. Pull out the potatoes or rice if in the pot. Flip the rack To the low position if needed and place the pork tenderloin back in the Ninja Foodi.
- Pork cooked and ready to air fry
- Set the Ninja Foodi to Air Crisp on High for 10 minutes. Depending on how crispy you want the bacon, and how fatty it is you may need to cook longer.

Nutrition Info

Calories: 280 Total Fat: 8g Carbohydrates: 27g Protein: 23g

Cheesy Beef and Rice Casserole

Prep/Cook Time 30 mins, Servings: 8

Ingredients

- 2 cloves garlic chopped
- 1 and 1/2 cup frozen chopped spinach
- 3 cups rice
- 3 and 1/3 cups chicken broth you can substitute beef broth or water
- 1 and 1/2 pounds lean ground beef
- 1 cup shredded cheddar cheese
- 1/2 cup onions chopped
- 1/2 cup red bell pepper chopped
- 1/4 cup scallions chopped
- 1/4 cup shredded mozzarella cheese OPTIONAL
- 2 tablespoons canola or vegetable oil
- 1 teaspoon kosher salt
- 1/2 teaspoon ground pepper
- 1/2 teaspoon granulated garlic
- 1/2 teaspoon paprika

Instructions

- Set the Ninja Foodi to SAUTE and add oil
- add the chopped onion, pepper and green onion to the Foodi and saute for 5 minutes
- add ground beef, salt, pepper, garlic powder ane paprika then brown for 5 minutes then add garlic. Cook for 30 seconds more
- Stir in the rice then add chicken broth and frozen spinach
- Cover the Ninja Foodi with the pressure cook lid then cook on HIGH pressure for 3 minutes
- Natural release for 10 minutes then manually release the rest of the pressure
- Reserve 1/2 a cup of cheese for the top. Stir in the rest of the cheddar and mozzarella cheese.
- Top with reserved cheddar cheese then close the AIR CRISP LID. BROIL for about 5 minutes or until the cheese is melted and browned.

Nutrition Info

Calories: 186 Total Fat: 14g Saturated Fat: 6g Trans Fat: 0g

Ninja Foodi Grill Juicy Grilled Pork Chops

Prep/Cook Time 28 minutes, Servings: 4

Ingredients

- 4 Pork Chops, bone in or boneless
- Pork Marinade

Instructions

- Make the pork marinade in advance and get your pork chops marinating in the refrigerator before cooking.
- Insert removable cooking pot. Insert grill grate into your pot.
- Press grill button, set to high (500 degrees), set time to 15 minutes.
- Once "Add Food" flashes, add pork chops onto grill, close lid.and grill for 7-8 minutes, than flip the meat, closing grill once again. Cook for another 5 minutes and check internal temperature to see if has reached an internal temperature of 150 degrees.
- Allow meat to rest 5 minutes before cutting and serving.

Nutrition Info

Calories: 523, Total Fat: 32g, Saturated Fat: 8g, Sugar: 4g, Protein: 48g

Crispy Pork Carnitas

Prep/Cook Time 55 minutes, Servings 4 people

Ingredients

- 1/2 tsp oregano
- 1/2 tsp cumin
- 2 lbs pork butt chopped into 2 inch pieces
- 1 tsp kosher salt
- 1 orange cut in half
- 1 yellow onion peeled and cut in half
- 6 garlic cloves peeled and crushed
- 1/2 cup chicken broth

Instructions

- Place pork, salt, oregano, and cumin in Ninja Foodi pressure cook insert. Combine making sure the seasonings are covering the pork.
- Take the orange and squeeze the juices over the pork. Put the squeezed orange in the insert, along with the onion, garlic cloves, and ½ cup chicken broth.
- Cover the Ninja Foodi with the pressure cooker cover, ensuring the valve is set to seal. Set the Ninja Foodi to High Pressure and cook for 20 minutes.
- Once the 20 minute timer is complete, do a quick release by switching the valve to vent. Once all the pressure is released, open the lid and remove the orange, onion, and garlic cloves.
- Set the Ninja Foodi to satué and select md:hi. The liquid will begin to simmer. Allow the liquid to cook until it reduces, about 10-15 minutes.
- Once the majority of the liquid has reduced, press stop on the Ninja Foodi and then close the Ninja Foodi Air Crisp lid.
- Select Broil and adjust the time to 8 minutes.
- Once complete, use the crispy delicious meat in tacos, bowls, sandwiches, wraps, etc. Top with cilantro or any of your favorite toppings.

Nutrition Info

Calories: 335kcal, Carbohydrates: 8g, Protein: 43g, Fat: 13g, Saturated Fat: 4g, Cholesterol: 136mg, Sodium: 838mg, Potassium: 909mg, Fiber: 1g, Sugar: 4g

Quick Chili in the Ninja Foodi

Prep/Cook Time 28 mins, Servings: 10

Ingredients
- 1 green pepper
- 29 ounces fire roasted tomatoes 2 14.5 oz cans
- 1 Tbsp Cholula
- 6 oz tomato paste
- 1 jalepeno pepper
- 3 cups beef stock
- 1 1/2 lb top sirloin
- 1 1/2 lb ground beef
- 1 onion
- 3-4 cloves garlic minced. About 2-3 tsp.
- 32 ounces kidney beans canned

Seasoning Blend
- 1 Tbsp Sea Salt
- 1 Tbsp Smoked Paprika
- 2 Tbsp Chili Powder
- 2 Tbsp Cumin
- 1 1/2 tsp Black Pepper
- 1/2 tsp Chipotle

Instructions
- Dice up onion, jalapeno pepper, and green pepper. Mince garlic. Combine seasonings in a medium bowl.
- Turn the Ninja Foodi on High Saute and add in ground beef. Trim and cube the sirloin into 1/2" pieces. Add to the inner pot with onions and seasonings. Saute for 5 minutes.
- Add in the minced garlic and saute for 2 minutes or until the ground beef is 50%-75% done.
- Add in the green pepper, jalapeno pepper, Cholula, and beef broth. Use a plastic scraper to scrape along the bottom of the pot to make sure nothing has stuck to it.
- Add in the fire roasted tomatoes and do not stir. Place the tomato paste on top and do not stir. Put on the pressure cooker lid and make sure the valve is to seal. Set the pressure to high for 10 minutes.
- Allow to natural release for 3 minutes and then manually release the remaining pressure. Remove the lid and add in the kidney beans. Stir to incorporate. Now is a good time to give it a little taste to see if you want to add any more spice or seasoning. Close the Tender Crisp lid and allow to sit for 5 minutes to thicken. If you are not serving it right away, you can turn on the keep warm button with the pressure lid on vent.

Nutrition Info
Calories: 429kcal, Carbohydrates: 31g, Protein: 36g, Fat: 16g, Saturated Fat: 6g, Cholesterol: 88mg, Sodium: 1088mg

Air Fryer Pork Loin

Prep/Cook Time 25 minutes, Servings 8

Ingredients

- 1 tsp salt
- 2 lb pork loin
- 1 tsp garlic powder
- 1 tsp basil
- 3 tbsp brown sugar

Instructions

- Mix seasoning together and then press it on all sides of loin. Cutting it in half first will be necessary so it will fit into your basket.
- Put into air fryer basket, close. Set to 400 degrees for 8 minutes.
- Open and flip loins and cook for 10 more minutes or until internal temperature reaches 145 degrees. Allow to rest for 10 minutes before slicing to maintain juiciness.

Nutrition Info

Calories 168 Calories from Fat 45, Fat 5g, Saturated Fat 1g, Cholesterol 71mg, Sodium 348mg, Potassium 435mg, Carbohydrates 5g, Fiber 1g, Sugar 4g, Protein 25g

Air Fryer Ninja Foodi Steak

Prep/Cook Time: 22 minutes, Servings: 1

Ingredients

- Celtic sea salt
- pepper
- filet mignon
- avocado oil

Instructions

- Lightly spray steak with oil
- salt and pepper to taste
- place your steak on high rack
- select air crisp on ninja foodi
- set temp at 375
- set time for 17 minutes
- flip steak over at halfway point

Nutrition Info

Calories: 162 Total Fat: 2g Saturated Fat: 1g Trans Fat: 0g Unsaturated Fat: 1g Cholesterol: 49mg Sodium: 411mg Carbohydrates: 25g

Keto Ninja Foodi Pressure Cooker Pulled Pork

Prep/Cook Time: 2 hrs 13 mins, Servings: 4

Ingredients

- 2 tsp Natural Sea Salt
- 1 tsp Black Pepper
- 1 tsp Smoked Paprika
- 3 lb Boneless Pork Roast, frozen or fresh - if using frozen, the machine will simply take a longer time to come to pressure. No other adjustments needed
- 1 cup Chicken Bone Broth, I used Mushroom Chicken Bone Broth because that's what I had but regular chicken is awesome
- 1 tsp Garlic Powder
- 1/2 tsp Red Pepper Flakes
- 3/4 cup Sugar-Free BBQ Sauce

Instructions

- Add the frozen or fresh roast, bone broth and seasonings to the removable cooking pot
- Close the Pressure Lid, turn the valve to "SEAL" and set the Ninja Foodi Pressure Cooker to "Pressure Cook". It'll take about 10 minutes to come to pressure since the meat is frozen. If you're using fresh meat, then it will come to pressure sooner. No other adjustments needed.
- Set the time to 90 minutes or 1 hour and 30 minutes and press "Start/Stop"
- Set the valve to "Vent" for a quick release of the air. Once the steam finishes escaping. Open the pressure lid.
- Remove the roast from the pressure cooker and shred the meat with meat claws or two forks
- Turn the Ninja Foodi to "Sear/Saute" and allow the cooking broth to come to a rolling boil/bubble.
- Mix in the BBQ sauce and allow it to reduce by half (~5 minutes).
- Mix in the shredded meat to the cooker and turn the Ninja Foodi off.

Nutrition Info

Calories 268 Calories from Fat 63, Fat 7g, Saturated Fat 2g, Cholesterol 119mg, Sodium 1075mg, Potassium 720mg, Carbohydrates 2g, Protein 43g

SNACKS AND APPETIZERS RECIPES

Ninja foodi french toast casserole

Prep/Cook Time: 25 minutes, Servings: 6

Ingredients

- 2 packs Grands cinnamon rolls
- 4 eggs
- 1 tbs vanilla
- 2 tbs milk
- 1 tbs cinnamon

Instructions

- whisk together eggs, milk, vanilla
- Open the grands cinnamon rolls and quarter each dough Put aside the icing
- Spray insert to the Ninja foodi with Pam or cooking oil.
- Place dough in the pan, pour over the egg mixture.
- Place Ninja Foodi on bake for 350 close air fry lid and bake for 20 minutes.
- Top with Syrup or icing from rolls

Nutrition Info

Calories: 161 Total Fat: 6g Saturated Fat: 2g Trans Fat: 0g Unsaturated Fat: 3g Cholesterol: 124mg Sodium: 229mg Carbohydrates: 20g Fiber: 1g Sugar: 8g Protein: 6g

Air Fryer Boxed Brownies

Prep Time: 5 mins , Cook Time: 30 mins, Servings: 18

Ingredients

- 1 box brownie mix prepared
- 1 tbsp butter softened

Instructions

- Butter two air fryer spring-form or cake barrel pans well and set aside.
- Prepare brownie mix according to package instructions and then divide into the two pans.
- One batch at a time, place the pan down into the air fryer basket and air fry at 300 for 30 minutes. If using the Ninja Foodi, use the air crisp feature.
- Check brownie center for doneness and bake for additional time if needed.
- Carefully remove pan from air fryer and cool before cutting brownies into portions.
- Repeat steps with second batch.

Nutrition Info

Calories: 131kcal, Carbohydrates: 22g, Protein: 1g, Fat: 4g, Saturated Fat: 1g, Cholesterol: 2mg, Sodium: 88mg, Sugar: 14g

Classic Sour Cream Coffee Cake & Ninja Coffee

Prep/Cook Time: 43 mins, Servings: 12-15 slices

Ingredients

For the cake

- 1 cup unsalted butter, softened
- 2 cups granulated sugar
- 2 large eggs
- 1 cup light sour cream
- ½ teaspoon vanilla extract
- 2 cups all-purpose flour, sifted
- 2 teaspoons baking powder
- ¼ teaspoon salt
- For the streusel
- 4 tablespoons unsalted butter, melted
- ½ cup light brown sugar, packed
- ½ cup + 2 tablespoons all-purpose flour
- 1 tablespoons cinnamon
- ½ cup pecans, chopped
- For the glaze:
- 1 cup powdered sugar
- 2 tablespoons heavy whipping cream (or milk)
- 1 teaspoon vanilla extract
- 2 teaspoons lemon juice (optional)

Instructions

- Preheat oven to 350°F.
- Allow butter to come to room temperature or microwave for 10-15 seconds. Cream butter and sugar together in a stand mixer until light and fluffy, about 3-4 minutes.
- Add eggs into batter and beat until well incorporated, scrape down the sides of the bowl.
- Next, add sour cream and vanilla extract and beat until well incorporated.
- In a separate bowl, sift flour (sifting is optional but recommended) and combine with baking powder and salt. Slowly had the flour and beat at a low speed just until flour is mixed. Turn off your mixer and use a spatula and mix by hand until well combined. Make sure to turn the batter from the bottom to the top to ensure it is well mixed.
- To prepare the streusel, melt butter in a microwave-safe bowl for 30 seconds. Combine butter with all dry ingredients. Mix together until well blended. Add chopped pecans.
- Spray the bottom of a 9-inch by 13-inch pan. Pour 2/3 of the batter into the bottom of the pan and spread evenly. Then sprinkle half of the streusel over the batter. Top with remaining batter and streusel.
- Bake at 350°F for 32-35 minutes. Check the coffee cake for doneness by inserting a toothpick into the center of the cake. If the toothpick comes out clean, then the cake is done. Allow to cool completely.
- To prepare the glaze, Sift powerded sugar into a bowl. This step is necessary to create a smooth glaze. Add heavy cream (or milk) and vanilla extract and stir to combine. Mixture will be thick.
- SLOWLY squeeze in the lemon juice and mix to cut the sweetness until desired taste.
- For a thicker glaze, add only 1 tablespoon of milk instead of 2. Or add additional powdered sugar. There is no secret to the glaze, you have to alternate milk and powdered sugar until desired consistency and taste.

Nutrition Info

Calories: 160 Total Fat: 7g Saturated Fat: 6g Trans Fat: 0g, Cholesterol: 94mg

Crème brûlée

Prep/Cook Time 35 minutes, Servings: 4

Ingredients
- 600 ml di fresh cream
- 6 egg yolks
- 120 g of caster sugar
- 2 tablespoons of instant coffee
- 10 cardamom pods
- cane sugar

Instructions
- The night before. Crush the cardamom pods in a mortar and put them to infuse into the cream. Leave to infuse in the fridge overnight.
- The day after. Filter cream removing the cardamom pods and heat over medium heat, when it begins to simmer add the instant coffee, stir until it is completely melted, remove from heat and let cool.
- Beat the egg yolks with sugar in a bowl. Pour over the cream and mix throughly, then bring back to the heat stirring constantly with a wooden spoon, when the egg mixture begins to thicken and veils the back of the spoon remove from heat (do not overcook otherwise you'll have scrambled eggs!).
- Pour in the custard into individual ramekins and put them in a large baking pan with 3 inches of water. Cook in preheated oven to 160°C for about 25 minutes, until it gets firm. Remove from heat, let cool completely and store in the fridge.
- Just before serving, sprinkle with cane sugar, caramelise the surface with a gas torchand serve immediately... enjoy!

Nutrition Info
Calories: 134kcal, Carbohydrates: 20g, Protein: 14g, Fat: 7g, Saturated Fat: 2g

Ninja Foodi Cake

Prep/Cook Time 38 minutes, Servings 6

Ingredients
- 1 box cake mix we used carrot cake boxed cake + ingredients to make batter as directed

Instructions
- Pour 1.5 c water into your Ninja Foodi. Lower down a trivet, I like one with handles.
- Prepare cake mix as directed. Spray non stick spray into your 7" bundt pan and pour your batter in, not more than 3/4 of the way full. It will fit an entire prepared box of cake.
- Cover bundt pan with foil.
- Put bundt pan on the trivet inside the pot.
- Close your pressure cooker lid, one that isn't attached. Close steam valve.
- Turn pot on, then push pressure button. Set to high for 28 minutes. When done allow steam to naturally release.
- Then lift out pan and take off the foil immediately and allow to cool in pan.
- Then put a plate on top and gently flip over, cake should fall out easily (that's when the non stick spray will come in handy).
- Warm frosting and pour on top. Slice and serve.

Nutrition Info
Calories 317 Calories from Fat 18, Fat 2g Saturated Fat 1g, Sodium 627mg, Potassium 40mg, Carbohydrates 71g, Fiber 1g, Sugar 37g, Protein 3g

CPSIA information can be obtained
at www.ICGtesting.com
Printed in the USA
LVHW021230201220
674641LV00011B/493